Things They Never Taught In Massage School

Nina Ward

ISBN: 9798620393572

Dedication

For Angel, my fellow Massage Therapist and friend.
We shared hundreds of stories about life as a massage therapist.
This is what kept us sane and in business

FORWARD

There are things you never learn in massage school. As you read these stories, feel free to laugh, learn, and love your job even in the most uncomfortable circumstance. I wrote this guidebook to give fellow massage therapists and other body-workers a resource to use when they aren't sure how to handle an awkward situation. And to reassure that you are not alone.

Massage therapists train to keep a sterile environment, good business skills, and the massage at a steady flow. When things don't go as expected, sometimes feelings of inadequacy or anger will evolve. You might wonder if you could have prevented the situation.

Most times it's a ridiculous scenario you just have to laugh at. These experiences do not happen often, but when they do, my hope as an author is for you to find help, comfort, and laughter.

I also hope others, not in the industry will get a glimpse and a giggle into the real world of massage therapy.

This is a compilation of stories I've gathered over twenty years in the industry from practitioners all over the United States who share their experiences, knowledge, and helpful tips. I don't mention the location or name of therapists and clients to protect the innocent, not so innocent, and immensely embarrassed.

Massage therapists have a rewarding career with little stress.

We love helping clients reduce pain, relieve stress, and maintain health, but sometimes crap happens. This brings me to our first scenario. You'll see why. Read on.

Oh Crap!

My first appointment of the day was a silver-haired elderly Caucasian woman seeking help to reduce lower back pain. This was her second visit to my facility. I started her prone so I could work the entire back and get deep into the Gluteus Maximus and all the buttock muscles to release the tension on the low back area.

After releasing the scapula and using other modalities, it was time to give the back a break and move to the glutes. I removed the sheet draped across her bare buttocks. I had my bag of tricks for working on back issues and it was going smoothly. Too, smoothly.

'Hmm,' I thought. *I don't remember seeing freckles on her arms or face, but there's a wicked amount of freckles on her buttocks!*

I thought nothing of it. It's hard to recall everyone's detailed anatomy, so I continued happily on. I added more lotion to my hands and began to warm the gluteal muscles with medium pressure strokes gliding up the back of the hamstrings over the buttocks to the middle of the back. And just like magic, those freckles disappeared!

These were definitely not freckles. Take a guess.

Yes, it most likely was from a recent bowel movement and the poor woman had no idea she missed a few spots when cleaning. And this poor massage therapist, me, had no clue as what to do but instantly throw up my contaminated hands and assess the situation as quickly as possible.

Things I considered
- Do you excuse yourself and wash your hands?

- What is your excuse for breaking the flow of the massage and leaving the room?

- How do you explain what just happened without embarrassing your client?

- How do you get rid of the now spread out freckled mess? Or do you?

What I Did

I thanked God I had the luxury of a sink directly behind me with towels stacked on the counter. I quickly washed my hands and forearms, grabbed a steamed towel from the towel cabinet, and mumbled something to my client about using a towel to soften the pressure so it wouldn't hurt.

My client didn't even hear me. She was a bit deaf. And she had fallen asleep!

What Not to Do
- The instant you notice the situation, try to refrain from shouting "Yuck" or "That's disgusting."

- These type of words or phrases should not come out of your mouth. It's a good idea to keep your thoughts in your head.

- Do not gag. At least try not to gag.

- Do not continue to spread the mixture of oil an "freckles" on any more parts of the client's body.

- Do not worry about breaking the flow of the massage.

TIPS

- If you have a steamed towel cabinet or anything nearby to cleanse your hands, then you are in luck. It is better to break the massage flow than to continue.

- Use a warm or steamed towel and tell your client you will use a heated towel to loosen the muscles. If you have a microwave, you can dampen a small towel and microwave for 1-2 minutes. Or run under hot water from a sink. Always test the temperature of the heated towel. If the towel is too hot, shake it to cool down. Everyone's body is different; it's a good idea to ask the client if they are comfortable with the temperature of the towel.

- Keep a spray bottle filled with water and a washcloth nearby for any future situations that need cleansing.

- This might be a good time to invest in a hot towel cabinet if you don't own one. Steamed towels also work well on stinky feet. You can add heated towels as an extra charge or a complimentary service. As a complimentary service, most client's will feel special and spoiled. It can be the tie-breaker for going to another facility where they do not treat clients with such personal care.

- Most clients love and appreciate a hot towel service. It

not only causes the mind to calm, it also warms and relaxes the muscles, making those rock-hard muscles easier to work with. Using heated towels also gives the therapist a break from deep physical work.

The Search for the Missing Eye

This was the longest scalp massage probably ever performed. At least it felt that way. My client was an elderly woman with tightly permed curls in a short hair-style. She was lying on her stomach, becoming more and more relaxed as I massaged the scalp. Then it happened. My glass eye fell into her hair! Popped right out like a rabbit out of its hole looking for a free meal in the garden.

I don't know why some people still call it a glass eye, because nowadays it is constructed of hard plastic acrylic, painted to look like the iris and pupil of the other eye. It's not really an eye. Vision doesn't exist. It covers the structures in the eye socket, similar to a contact lens covering the pupil. Still, I'm sure it would not please this woman to know an eyeball was lost in her head.

My mind began to panic while searching for the shell-shaped prosthesis in the web of curls. Simultaneously as I searched, I worried what to do when I found it. My eye patch was at home. I did not want this woman to look into a face with an empty eye socket. That would kill the effects of the massage real quick. Either way, I would have to excuse myself to clean and put the eye back in.

With one hand, I massaged the scalp. With the other, I tediously ran my fingers through the curls as if I was mining for gold, but the white part of the eye blended in with her white hair. I wondered if it might have fallen on the sheet or on the floor. By the time that thought crossed my mind, my client looked up to let me know she felt a little dizzy. I checked to see if I saw anything roll out of her head. Nope, no runaway eyeballs! I was about to give up when I saw it stuck at the bottom of her neck.

Things I Considered
- Do I wait till the end of the massage and hope she doesn't look up before I leave the room?

- What if I can't find the lost item? How long should I keep searching?

- What if it rolls off the sheet onto the floor, and she crushes it with her feet when she gets off the table to get dressed? What if it gets caught between her toes?

- If my client happens to look up, I'd have to explain an empty eye socket. She might think I am winking at her, but I am trying to keep the eyelid shut. I don't want her to think I was *giving her the eye* and am attracted to her!

What I Did

After I secured the prosthesis, I tried to keep the eyelid closed and explained "I'm sorry, I'm having trouble with my eye prosthesis. Excuse me, I'll be right back. When I returned, I thanked her for waiting. To show my appreciation, I asked her if she would like a complimentary extra ten minutes added to her session.

What Not to Do
- Do not grab the following items to create a makeshift eye-patch: Sports bra, medical face mask, pillowcase.

- Try not to allow the client to see the opened eye socket.

- Do not say any of the following aloud: 'Well that's a first.' Your client will ask, "What's a first?" You don't want to answer that question.

- In your frustration searching for the lost item, do not say, "Where the *&^%$ is my eye?"

TIPS
- Try to keep the eye shut. If you keep winking, In a light-hearted way inform your client you're not making sexual advances by winking. Explain how you're trying to keep the eyelid shut so she won't become alarmed if she sees an empty eye socket.

- There's nothing left to do now except be honest and explain the situation.

- If you don't have the time in-between clients, offer extra time with their next massage or knock off a few dollars for the session.

- Keep five or ten-dollar gift certificates handy for times like these. If you can't make up time lost in the current session, offer a gift certificate for the next appointment. Customers love gift certificates and feel special when presented with one.

- Be honest. Be real. Similar situations can occur such as when a client or therapist passes gas. Circumstantial evidence such as noise or smell leaves no other alternative except to give an honest response.

Breast Attack

Many people who suffer from obesity never receive a professional massage because they fear their weight will cause problems. They're afraid they won't fit on the table or the table won't hold their weight. Most are insecure and embarrassed about their bodies. So when someone with the issue of obesity schedules an appointment, I am happy they feel comfortable enough with me to relax and get the massage therapy they desperately need.

One of those type of clients was a big-breasted, stunning woman of 30, huge brown eyes to go along with a big heart and body-easily 250 pounds. This was her first massage experience, and I wanted to make her feel comfortable and secure. The massage room provides a safe, nonjudgmental environment. I did not know how large she was until she walked in.

She asked the usual question, "Will I break the table?"

"Are you more than 500 pounds?" I jokingly asked. "The table has only a 500-pound limit."

I realized immediately she might not know I was joking. My comment wasn't meant to assume she was 500 pounds, so I quickly added "You have nothing to worry about."

When I walked into the room, she fumbled with the twin sheet as she tried to cover her body that overflowed off the side of the table. She asked me if I could massage a scar on her abdomen from a recent surgery. I grabbed a medium sized towel to cover her chest knowing the towel would only cover three-quarters of what needed to be covered, but it was all I had.

New clients must fill out a health intake form and this is when she relayed to me how she was on a mission to lose weight because of a health scare. She hired a nutritionist and fitness trainer at a local gym. It was her trainer who suggested massage to help with the scar tissue and weight she wanted to drop. The only thing dropped on that first fateful day on the massage table was her breast.

******

My client lay supine under the twin sheet with both hands clasped to hold her arms on her chest. I don't think an armrest table extender would have been any help, but it was now added to my supply list of business equipment to purchase.

With the towel secured in one hand, I gently but swiftly pulled the sheet off her chest to uncover the stomach to begin work. With a large breasted woman, without a bath-sized towel, this process of keeping the client covered is like trying to keep a hat on a baby's head. Not going to happen.

After a soothing facial and neck massage, I was ready to loosen the shoulder and neck muscles. Slowly and rhythmically, I took her left arm to begin a range of motion stretches. The music in the background played softly.

"This feels so good," my client whispered as I pulled the arm down along her hip. I began gently to lift the arm out to her side. If you can imagine in slow motion, the breast flopped out of the towel off the side of the table, knocked my ninety-five-pound petite body and pushed me slightly off my feet. The breast then lay limp off the table, hanging like a piece of fresh-butchered meat.

As soon as I was confident I was not harmed by the breast attack, I assessed the situation. The breast, although not the largest breast in the world, had to weigh at least fifteen pounds which meant I needed two hands to maneuver the part back in place. At this point, I remembered reading of the largest breasts in the world owned by Annie Hawkins. In the year 2000 she made it into the Guinness Book of World Records with each breast weighing in at about fifty-six pounds.[1] Somehow this made me feel better. I was glad this client was not Annie.

The breast, stared back at me and seemed to say, "So you gonna leave me hanging or what? What ya gonna do with me?"

Things I Considered
- Do I put the breast back?

- If I put the breast back in its proper place, how do I handle that transition?

- Do I ask the client to take care of the situation?

What I Did

I glanced to see if my client had even noticed. She did. I looked at her. I looked at the breast. I looked at her again and asked, "Do you want me to put that back or do you want to take care of it?" Thankfully, she put it back.

Later that week, I bought table extenders, a bath-sized towel and flat queen sheets to keep on hand. I have not lost a breast, since!

What Not to Do
- Do not try to catch the breast and save it from falling

- Do not try to secure the breast by throwing it over the client's shoulder and hope it will stay in place.

- Do not touch the breast without asking the client.

TIPS

- Purchase an armrest extender for your massage table.

- Keep a few large sheets and large towels on hand.

- Always ask the client for permission to touch the chest area.

---

[1] https://www.thetalko.com/15-women-with-the-biggest-cup-sizes-in-the-world/

The Many Facets of Farts

My first client for the morning was a petite eighty-year-old female being treated by her physician for low back and tailbone issues without much success. The physician recommended massage to manage her pain. When it was time to turn her over onto her stomach, I asked her how she was doing.

"I'm wonderful," she said. "Just wonderful. I'm so relaxed."

Less than five minutes after she was prone, I heard the classic sounds of passing gas. It happens. When one is in a state of total relaxation, this is a normal reaction. Of course, I was in the direct vicinity of this eruption. The air from the outgoing gas was so strong that the sheet lifted a few inches. I swear this to be true. The odor was rank. It took everything in me not to gag. When the effects from one lingering fart seemed to die, another emitted slow and heavy. I couldn't be sure I would last another twenty-five minutes until the end of the massage, especially if more was to come.

Several things go through your mind at once when a client passes gas. Your main goal is to survive. Your second goal is to keep the client from being embarrassed. Keeping the client from being embarrassed is not going to happen unless they sleep through the incident. It is what it is. You fart in public and you are embarrassed.

I couldn't understand how this pint-sized lady could do so much damage to the environment.

Things I Considered
- Do I need to leave the area and continue on to another part of the body perhaps as far away as possible?

- Will the air be filled with more unpleasant odors?

- Does the client know what happened?

What I Did

With a swift turn to the opposite side of the table, I moved out of the danger zone.. Two additional toots were heard but not seen. They were definitely felt. I thought I was going to choke if the air didn't start to clear. With my left hand, I grabbed a nearby bottle of peppermint oil and rested my right forearm between the scapulas (shoulder blades) in order to free my hands to dab the oil on my wrist and temple. This covered up the foul scent. My client, who was fully awake but totally relaxed, did not acknowledge the fart, nor did I.

What Not to Do
- Do not use an air freshener spray to saturate the room. This will only cause both client and therapist to choke on cheap fragrance.

- Do not cover your nose with your hands to avoid the stench. This is for obvious health reasons. Unless you want to do a one-handed massage until the air clears and get oil or lotion all over your face-don't cover your nose.

- If your initial reflex causes you to grab the sheet off the client to cover your face from the horrific odors, place the sheet back as quick as possible and don't do it again. Apologize and be honest. Let the client know you were intoxicated from the gas.

TIPS

- Keep a spray bottle mixed with essential oil and water to freshen the air. Spray in moderation. A little usually goes a long way. Make sure your client has no known sensitivities to essential oils.

- Keep a medical face-mask handy to cover your nose and mouth. Don't worry about offending the client. If you start to gag, you're probably going to offend them, anyway. You can always say you're wearing a mask because of a weakened immune system.

- Turn a fan on if available.

- Keep a humidifier or diffuser with a mist that sprays essential oils.

Wipeout!

It was fashionable in the 1940s for women to shave their eyebrows and pencil them in with thin strokes. Unfortunately, some eyebrows never grew back. It never dawned on me that this can happen to the women of today until I swiped an eyebrow off a client's face.

With my hands full of lotion, I soothed the facial muscles above the left eyelid with long sweeping strokes. The eyebrow disappeared as quickly as a chocolate-chip cookie in the hands of a child. It happened at the beginning of the facial massage so I had time to consider how to remedy the situation. My first thought was, 'How can I put it back?'

Things I Considered
- Do I leave the lone eyebrow without a partner?

- How can I create a new eyebrow? If I had an eyebrow pencil, I could cough and tell my client, "I must be allergic to your hair products. Excuse me, I'll get a cough drop." I'd come back with the pencil and sneak the new eyebrow on the face by alternating massage strokes and pencil strokes. I'd have to match the other eyebrow with the same color, but I didn't own an eyebrow pencil. I filed this complicated idea and made a note to myself to purchase a variety of colored eyebrow pencils in case of another occurrence.

- Should I wipe the other eyebrow off for balance?

What I Did

After I envisioned my client stopping at the store on her way home, wondering why everyone was staring, I wiped the other eyebrow off the face. I apologized and explained to my client what happened. Trying to lighten the mishap, I joked, "I took off your other eyebrow since it was smeared anyway and I don't want you to walk out of the massage unbalanced."

"According to my psychologist I have a long way to go till I'm balanced," she joked. At least I thought she was joking.

What Not to Do

- Don't become verbally alarmed or gasp when you first notice the missing eyebrow.

- Don't grab a marker or crayon and try to fix the problem.

- Don't withhold information about the missing eyebrow. If the client is stopping at another location after their massage appointment, they will want to know. Not all clients check themselves in the mirror before they leave.

TIPS

- Don't assume all eyebrows are real.

- Remain calm.

- Always be cautious around and on the eyebrow area if using oils or lotions.

Sleeping Beauty

It is a compliment to the massage therapist when a client falls asleep on the table. It means they have received a relaxing massage they desperately needed from skilled hands. But what happens when they don't wake up?

During this one hour massage my client's limp body fell in and out of a quick sleep several times.

To let the client know the session had ended, I placed my hand on his back. "You're all set. I hope you're feeling better. Take your time and when you're dressed, come out to the waiting area."

He never came out.

After I washed up and finished the client's SOAP notes (medical data), an office mate from next door stopped in to chat. Since my next client's appointment was two hours away, I welcomed the company to fill the time, even though there was plenty of business stuff to do. Chatting seemed like much more fun!

Twenty-five minutes flew by, and it wasn't until then that I realized my client never came out of the room. This was an elderly gentleman and my first thought was, 'Is he alive?'

Come to think about it, he didn't respond or move when I patted him on the back and announced the session had ended.

The two-room office is small with walls thin enough to carry on a conversation with my neighbor on the other side. If he was asleep, he would have awakened by the chatter and passing fire-truck sirens.

I was afraid to open the door. What if he passed away? I knocked lightly and called his name. No response. I knocked harder. Nothing. I banged and shouted. Still, no response.

Things I Considered

- There was only one entrance to my office so he couldn't have exited out a back door without paying - a thought that crossed my mind.

- My brain led me to places I did not want to go. Did he die from a heart attack? Am I going to jail for killing a client?

What I Did

With a cell phone in hand, in case I had to call 911, I whisked enough courage to open the door. The man was dead asleep. I shook his shoulders and called his name to awaken him. He budged slightly. I pushed harder. He moved to turn his head. Finally, I gave the shoulders a two-second kneading and used tapotement to chop alongside the spine. The short rapid chops from my hands stirred him enough to waken. He apologized and explained he suffered from insomnia, something he forgot to let me know during his session.

What Not to Do

- Never forget you have a client in the session room.

- Don't turn up the volume to the relaxation music. It won't work. Sounds of waves, animals, rain, or soothing instrumentals can't increase the volume high enough to awaken anyone.

TIPS
- Pat yourself on the back for a job well done!
  You've helped someone find relief from insomnia.

Drip Drop

The long, effleurage strokes sweep up and down on a well-oiled back as they dance to the music placing your client into a relaxation blitz. You, the therapist, are in sync with the intoxicating rhythm, also feeling the effects of the sounds and movements of the atmosphere.

Then, like a volcano erupting, you sense the slow flow of nasal drip streaming downward. You wonder how much time left until it drips out your nose, onto your lip or even worse-on the client's body. There's no denying a fountain of drips will speed towards the light to emerge every three minutes. Your eyes wander around the room to find the closest tissue or towel, but there are none in sight. The tissue box sits on a table in the dressing area on the other side of the room behind the room divider. The towels are folded in the cabinet outside the massage room. The only sheets in sight are the ones on your client.

Time is ticking. How do you stop the drip from landing on the client?

Things I Considered
- I could inconspicuously wipe my nose on my shirt.

- I could try to stop the leak by sniffling.

- I thought of wearing a disposable face-mask to catch the drips. I store pleated masks in my office for times when there is a slight chance a client or myself could be contagious.

What I Did

By the time I decided to take action, a drip or two fell downward to who knows where. All I know, it didn't land on me! As soon as I felt another drip, I'm sorry to say, my instantaneous reaction was to wipe with my shirt. But how long could I keep this up? It distracted me from applying the techniques I needed to apply to give this client the massage they needed. I interchangeably sniffled and wiped.

Things intensified when I sat at the client's feet to work reflexology points. My eyes began to tear and my nose ran faster than a cheetah, one of the fastest mammals on earth. This was not because of foot odor! The peppermint foot lotion, along with the air conditioner vent directly above my head, triggered the nasal drip. I could not continue using my already saturated shirt. I explained to my client, my sniffling was not because of a crack habit and excused myself to grab some tissues and wash my hands.

What Not to Do

- Don't try to sniffle the entire session. You can end up sniffling every five minutes for the full hour massage.

- Don't ignore the problem. If your sinus is draining down your throat, you could choke on the mucus.

TIPS

- Keep a box of tissues within reach of the table.

Spider Man

It was time to turn Mr. Marino to a prone position to finish the one-hour massage session. When I rolled the sheet down his back, I saw what looked like a common brown widow spider on the left side below the shoulder blade.

Although spiders are nature's best pest controllers, as they feed on insects we don't want around, I don't need a spider working in my office. There was a good chance Mr. Marino would never come around again if he knew a spider rested on his back.

In the moment, I knew I had to destroy and kill. These spiders are not aggressive so I wasn't afraid of being bit.

On this sunshiny cool autumn day I was more concerned with how the spider got into my office and if he brought any friends or relatives. Maybe the spider sought shelter from the cooler weather. This time of season, male spiders go indoors to hunt for a mate Hopefully this wasn't a male looking for some action!

Things I considered:

- I was ready to take a steamed towel out of the hot towel cabinet and place it on Mr. Marino's back. The spider would never survive the heat or my hands massaging over the towel. I'd simply wipe the smashed intruder off with the towel.

What I Did

In the dim lit room, I raised one hand up to smack and destroy with my weapon of choice-my hand loaded with tapotement chops.

There was nothing to worry about. The spider turned out to be one big brown hairy mole. When Mr. Marino left my office, I scheduled an appointment for an eye exam!

What Not to Do

- Do not yell "Yuck, a spider!

- Do not spray your client with a can of bug repellant or wasp killer.

TIPS

- If you spot an insect crawling under the massage table, try to smash it with your foot. You don't want your client to see bugs. It might creep them out or they might assume the office is infested and unhealthy.

Ghost

A first-time client comes in for a massage. Before I leave the room so that he can undress in private, I give him the basic instructions.

"Lay face up and cover up with the sheet and I will knock before I enter."

When I entered the room, he did exactly what was told; he covered his entire body, from head to toe with the sheet. Face and all.

I had an urge to jerk the covers off his face and yell, "Boo" !

Things I considered:

- Are we playing hide and seek?

- What kind of place does he think this is?

What I Did

I mustered up as much professionalism as possible and lowered the sheet off of his face, trying not to burst out in laughter.

What Not to Do

- Don't leave the sheet on the client's face.

TIPS

- Make a note on the client's SOAP notes that this client might be completely under the sheet the next time he prepares for his massage. On his next visit, try to explain clearly how to cover with the sheet. Example: Lie on your back, cover up with the sheet but KEEP YOUR FACE uncovered.

Snoring Thunder

She warned me. The warning was in writing on her intake form, under 'Are there any concerns or medical conditions the therapists should know about?'

She answered, "I snore during a massage."

Forty-five percent of adults snore. Not a big deal. It wasn't the first client who snored during a massage, and it wouldn't be the last.

But this lady was loud! Like scary thunderstorm loud throughout the entire massage. It eluded me how this woman could sleep through the noise.

Sporadic snores jarred me into oblivion with each eruption. It was difficult to create a relaxed atmosphere and maintain focus to work the needed areas of concern.

When the massage session ended, I called her name, nudging her to awake. Her eyes opened, she pasted a contented smile on her face, and asked, "Did I snore?"

Things I Considered

- If I had earplugs, I would have used them.

- To keep my client awake, I thought to apply hard tapotement chops every ten minutes.

- Lying on your side can prevent snoring if it is a tongue

issue. This makes the base of the tongue and soft palate collapse. I considered doing the entire massage with the client lying on her side.

What I Did

I spent most of the massage trying to stop the snoring. At first I tried using invigorating modalities like quick percussion or skin rolling. Striking my client with the side of my hand or stretching the skin to roll down the vertebrae did nothing except cause an increase in the volume level of the snore. My client insisted on falling in and out of a sleep with bursts of snoring whether she was on her back, side, or supine. It was funny at first but soon became annoying.

I wasn't aware of any issue that might cause the snoring, so my first guess was blocked nasal passages. Rubbing peppermint oil on her neck did not help.

I increased the volume on the relaxation music playing in the background, hoping the noise would keep her semi-conscious, but she was out cold most of the hour. Between the loud music and obnoxious snoring, my head started to throb within the last fifteen minutes of the massage. When she asked if she snored, I didn't hesitate to reply politely, "You bet!"

What Not to Do

- Do not be tempted to grab a cup of coffee and a good book and let the client sleep the entire hour.

- Do not use a Snore Stop Extinguisher on your sleeping client. Do not use without permission on a client who is awake; make sure each snoring client has their own personal extinguisher. You might suggest to your client to try this product at home. Yes, there really is a Snore Stop Extinguisher.

TIPS

- If snoring interferes with sleep, it could indicate sleep apnea or breathing issues. Refer your client to a physician.

- Try rubbing the neck or upper chest with coconut, peppermint or eucalyptus oil. Always check for any contraindications when using essential oils.

- If the nasal cavity is blocked, suggest to the client to use a nasal irrigation system such as a neti-pot.

- A self-help tip for your snoring client is to use herbs before going to sleep. Herbs that will open airways are thyme, licorice root, or ginger. Always check for any contraindications when using essential oils.

- Create a self-help take-home paper to offer to your clients.

Here's an example of a Self-Help Tip sheet:

Suggestions to Stop Snoring

Change your sleeping position. Sleep on your side. Keep trying to sleep sideways until it becomes a habit.

Elevate your head to breath easier. This will cause the jaw and tongue to stay forward.

Quit smoking. Smoking will irritate the membranes in your nose, throat, and mouth, which can block airways to breathe.

Use a humidifier to moisten the air. If your nasal passages are congested this will reduce swelling in your nasal tissues.

Use a mouth guard. Check with your dentist to see if you are a candidate for this device. There are also do-it-yourself kits available to purchase.

Increase vitamin C to 1000 milligrams a day. Taking vitamin C increases the immune system, which can reduce infections in the nasal cavity and throat. Snoring happens when the swelling from an infection block the nose and throat passageways.

Limit alcohol before bed if you suffer from sleep apnea. Alcohol disrupts your natural sleep patterns and causes you to breathe slower. Your throat muscles relax and can cause your upper airway to collapse that will cause snoring.

Avoid dairy and sugar. Dairy products can produce mucus.

Have a cup of peppermint tea to relieve congestion. Gargle with peppermint mouthwash.

Try Honey and Water to soothe a dry throat. Use one cup of warm water with one tablespoon of organic honey.

Tongue Exercises will strengthen weak throat and tongue muscles. Keep the tip of your tongue on the roof of your mouth and slide your tongue back. Repeat about 20 times.

Sock it! Try wearing compression stockings. Compression stockings allow the fluid in your legs to flow normally. It can keep fluid from traveling to your neck when you sleep.

Call a doctor if :
You snore loudly and suffer from fatigue during the day.
You gasp or choke in your sleep.
You fall asleep suddenly such as in the middle of a meal or conversation.

Boundaries

Every Thursday for two years, Mr. Browning scheduled an appointment for a deep-tissue and relaxation session. One summer morning when he was due to arrive in thirty minutes for his massage, I debated if I should cancel or make this his last appointment.

For the third time in two years, during his last visit, he used language that made me uncomfortable. He called me 'precious' during two different sessions. The first time, I ignored my gut feeling to say something. The second time, I politely asked him not to use those terms. He said he understood and wouldn't do it again. The third time, ten minutes into the session, he called me his 'teddy bear'. Again, I nicely asked him to refrain from that type of language.

Things I Considered

- My first gut feeling was to puke. Maybe then he'd realize how awful he made me feel.

- The very moment he called me 'teddy bear' I wanted to end the massage with a new technique called Fist Bump to the Head. This chopping motion wakes up muscles. In his case-the brain.

- I truly wanted to end the massage but summers are slow and I needed the money.

- I pondered whether I should make a big deal out of the situation. Did I want to lose this long time client that might never respect my boundaries?

- I became angry with myself because I should have been more affirmative when this client had his first session.

What I Did

I continued the massage seething with disgust and aggravation. When Mr. Browning's session ended, he came out of the room and happily paid for the services. "See you next week."

"I don't think so," I shot back.

I raised myself off the chair and stood tall, even though I am only five feet.

"Mr. Browning, I told you not to use certain language but you continue to disrespect my policies and boundaries. I am not the therapist for you. You'll have to find another therapist.

What Not to Do

- Don't be wishy-washy. The moment something makes you uncomfortable, stand your ground.

- Don't let anything slide, especially with a new client.

- Don't allow a client's behavior rob your peace of mind or steal the joy in what you do. It's not worth the money to deal with these type clients.

TIPS

- You can refer this type of client to a therapist of the opposite sex.

- Set your boundaries before you open your doors for business.

- The instant someone is not respecting your boundaries use a stern professional tone to warn them you will end the session if the behavior persists. Payment is not waived.

- If you have a scheduled client and decide you do not want to keep the appointment, be honest. Let them know you're sorry for the short notice, but you have to cancel the massage. Tell them you have strict client boundaries that have been disrespected and they need to find another therapist.

- Make sure all clients, new and existing understand your policies.

The Fight

Note to Self: Purchase several copies of the *Relaxation for Dummies* book. Sell these books to clients who do not understand the definition of the word *relax*. The sales would add a sizable income to my business!

Here's a typical scenario with a client who I'll call Cindy. Cindy has a stymied relaxation sensor. There are things in her life that have obstructed her ability to relax.

Therapist enters the room to begin the session.

Therapist: Hi, Cindy. How've you been? What's up with you, lately?

Cindy: (*Client is in a sitting position on the table, fidgeting with her phone*) What's up? My stress levels-that's what's up!

The Fight begins. Massage Therapist verses Client. The massage therapist must get the client to relax. The client must resist tightening their muscles; they must shut down their brain, and their mouth if they are talking incessantly.

There are heavyweight and lightweight clients who enter the massage room ring; some take forty-five minutes to finally relax and others may take fifteen. The heavyweights rarely find solace.

There are clients who believe with all their soul that they are totally relaxed. But when they are on the table, their shoulders are up to their ears and it's a fight to get them to loosen a limb to stretch a muscle.

There are clients who are continuously anxious and worried throughout the day and cannot turn off their mind. They seek massage therapy in hopes of relief. Some will talk during the entire massage. Sometimes people do need to vent, but it defeats the purpose of a relaxation massage if this is a constant event.

Massage therapists are sometimes like bartenders. People vent and we listen, maybe say an encouraging word or two. I used to have a client who came in three times a week. On Monday, she only wanted to talk. I felt like a psychiatrist as I sat in the chair, listening as my client lay supine on the table. Yes, I was paid to listen for the hour! On Wednesday and Friday she received a relaxation soft tissue massage.

So what can you pull up in your training to help these opponents lose their fight and give in to total relaxation?

Things I considered:
- To be honest, I want to hit them over the head with
  the *Relaxation for Dummies* book.

- If a client answers the phone during a massage, I
  want to snatch the phone out of their hands and throw
  the phone out the door.

- I considered permeating the room with high
  powered essential oils in the diffuser and in the lotion,
  then dab a drop straight out of the bottle under
  their nose, on the temple, and behind their neck.

What I Did

If I know a client has trouble relaxing, I will choose music that uses deep, intense meditation tones to induce a state of calmness. After my client takes a couple deep breaths, I like to start with a scalp massage to prompt calmness, then release the sub-occipital at the base of the occiput to soften the fascial tissue. Sometimes I have the client focus on their breathing to quiet their mind.

My tone of voice becomes softer and I offer words of serenity and hope if needed. I try to instill to the client that part of taking care of yourself is learning to relax so you can rejuvenate your mind and body. I acknowledge their effort to maintain their health through massage, especially when they are so busy. The time to relax is when you don't have time to relax!

What Not to Do

- Do not threaten your client with the following statement: *"If you came in for a relaxation massage, then you have to stop thinking and talking about your problems. If you don't relax, I'm going to sing and my voice is a lot worse than your problem!"*

- Don't overdose your client with Lang-Lang or Neroli oils to the point where they won't be able to get off the table at the end of the session.

- Beware of overdosing yourself with essential oils or aromas. I once fell asleep for a few seconds, maybe minutes, working reflexology on the feet.

TIPS

- Encourage your client to learn to relax. Suggest resources like yoga, music therapy, or Qi.gong. Keep a referral list or business cards of resources to hand out to clients. You can also negotiate a referral fee or incentive with other business'.

- Recommend books on the topic of relaxation, meditation, or finding peace.

- During the massage, use essential oils that promote calmness.

- If you don't already use music therapy in your practice, educate yourself on the benefits.

- Educate your client about aromatherapy. Make sure they understand the contraindication of using essential oils. Recommend oils that promote relaxation. Lang-Lang, lavender, sandalwood, and Neroli are a few oils to calm the body and mind.

- Offer your client a small cup of chamomile tea before session. Or suggest they drink a cup a half hour or more prior to their appointment.

"Your body is precious, as it houses your mind and spirit. Inner peace begins with a relaxed body.
Norman Vincent Peale

Circus Tent Man

It happens to all massage therapists sooner or later, especially female therapists. The dreaded moment when out of the corner of your eye, you spot the *tent*. The male client is supine and relaxed as the tent begins to rise. You continue to work the upper traps as the sheet covering his private parts rises to form a perfect Teepee tent. Does he know? "He must," you think to yourself. You look away, hoping the tent fell. No such luck. What do you do?

Once, a young married man received a gift
certificate from his wife for his first professional massage.
In the middle of his session, he realized his predicament.
He immediately sprang up, tried to cover himself,
and nervously commented, "How can this happen,
I wasn't even thinking anything sexual…"

I assured him he wasn't cheating on his wife and
even though this is a normal reaction, it doesn't mean
this will happen during each session. I wanted him
to continue seeking massage, a natural alternative to
maintain his health issues as opposed to his current plan
of heavy duty pain killers. Plus, I wanted his business!

Another time, early in my career, one of my
clients referred her brother to my office. He was new to
the area, and received regular massages. Although
he arrived uptight and stressed, he relaxed within

ten minutes on the table. I was hopeful he would be a consistent customer. Until I spotted the *tent*.

Things I Considered

- Maybe if I ignore the situation, it will go away.

- What do I do if it's time for my client to turn on his stomach and the tent is still erect?

- When I began work on the shoulders and arms, I thought of applying deep pressure, hoping the pain would distract attention away from situation.

What I Did

Just as deep as a politician's lies, I applied to the anterior delts and traps as much pressure as I could muster. Then I realized my client was submerged in a relaxation state and unaware of his heightened moments, so I ignored the issue. If he was behaving inappropriately, I would have terminated the session, collected my payment, and explained why. It took a few minutes for him to compose himself and eventually things went back to where they were before he got on the table.

What Not to Do

- Do not ignore any type of behavior that makes you feel uncomfortable. Be honest with yourself and to your client.

TIPS

- Over the course of your massage therapy career, there will be numerous times when a male client will have an erection. This can be a normal reaction for some. Unless they are behaving inappropriately, simply ignore.

- If a client becomes embarrassed, assure him this sometimes is a normal response to relaxation effects.

Quiet Please

In the middle of an intense massage session, the bell jingled to my three-room office as the front door opened, alerting me that someone had entered the waiting area. If I am in session and a client enters the front area, sometimes they will leave a note or wait till I am out of session. No one had ever knocked on the door to the massage room like a maniac until that day.

The knocks on the door to my massage room continued steady for what seemed like several minutes. There are two signs on the massage room door; A "Do not Disturb" sign hangs on the doorknob and a time card with the words "Quiet Please, Massage in Session" is clearly posted. The time card lets people know the time the session will be finished.

What part of the signs did the people on the other side of the door, not understand?

Things I considered:
- My first thought was the person knocking on the door was blind. No seeing person could walk into a business and be that rude or inconsiderate.

- My mind wandered to who might be behind the door; burglar, serial killer or worse, a salesperson! I made sure the door was locked. It was.

- I needed to communicate to the intruders to go away. I didn't want to break the flow of the massage, but then I didn't want to disturb the peaceful ambiance by shouting at them even though the pounding on the door caused disruption to the flow and quietness.

What I Did

When I realized the intruders were not going away, I didn't want to break the flow so I continued massaging and half shouted and half whispered, "Is this an emergency?"

"Can we tell you about God's good news?"

"Come back in a half hour and I'd be happy to hear about your faith and tell you about my relationship with God as a Christian believer."

They never came back.

What Not to Do
- I assumed if I didn't respond to the knocking they would go away. Never assume!

TIPS

- Post a 'Do Not Disturb" sign on the massage room door. If that doesn't work, pre-write on an index card any of the following notes below to slip under the door to the intruder :

*^Please do not knock on door or talk. This will induce
a violent emotional reaction to those behind this door.*

^Do not disturb means please go away.

*^Do not disturb unless there is an emergency involving
fire, water, or weather, or if you are giving away a
box of chocolate.*

Hands on Game

The Hands On game is common among older men and their massage therapist. It's played mostly by elderly widowers, but other senior citizens whether married or single have participated.

In my massage therapy practice, this game occurs at least two or more times during the course of a year and I loathe it each and every time. To give you an idea of how this game is played, here's a summary of what happened during the first time the Hands On Game debuted in my office.

Mr. Caruso, a gentleman of about seventy, came in to use his gift certificate for a one hour massage. I stood at the side of the table intensely working to loosen the left anterior deltoid. Suddenly, my client clutches my wrist and squeezes like he's holding on for dear life.

I was bewildered. I tried to interpret why he felt the need to do what he did.

Things I Considered
- My very first thought was that I hoped he wasn't pervert.

- I wanted to end the massage and yell,"What do you think

you're doing?

- I wondered if there was a motive or if it was an innocent reaction to touch.

What I Did

Immediately, I pulled my arm from the grip and stopped massaging, then scurried to the head of the table to work the neck. It didn't matter that I had already worked the area; I needed time to recover from the client clinging onto my hand.

A few minutes later I stood on the other side of the table. Once more he gripped my hand like he was clinging to the sides of a rollercoaster on its way down the track. With my free hand I unwrapped his hand from mine and explained, "Mr. Caruso, I do the touching. You don't."

"Oh, Oh, I'm so sorry. I don't even know why I did that," he said, what seemed to be like a sincere apology.

What Not to Do

- Don't make a big deal out of it.

- Don't grab him back and if you do, don't squeeze so hard that you fracture the bones in his hand.

- As much as you want to slap his hand or throw his arm off to the side-don't do it.

TIPS

- Try to be sensitive and professional.

- If the behavior makes you uncomfortable, decide if you will see this client in the future. If you don't want to keep this client as a customer, make sure he understands he will not be able to receive

massage sessions in your office if the behavior
continues. You might want to be honest and let him know
why you are uncomfortable.

Phone Addict

Through the years people have come through the doors of my therapeutic massage business to schedule a relaxation massage, but check or talk on their cell phone throughout the entire session. Then they wonder why their neck remains stiff and their headache still exists!

I had a high-powered celebrity client who came in to de-stress whenever he was in town. He arrived with a bodyguard who waited in the waiting area while my client received his hour and a half massage. During each session, my client would get on the table, take a deep breath, and tuck his phone under his right hip. He would answer the phone or make calls throughout the session. The conversations were mostly stressful and required his complete attention. I'd be working on his arms, the phone would ring and he'd break out of my grip to grab the phone. I'd be working on his back and he would suddenly lift his upper body to yell at the person on the other end of the phone line. It was extremely annoying.

Then there was Elizabeth, a fifty-five year-old mother and grandmother who could not be without a phone in her hand for more than one minute. She worried one of her kids or grandkids might need her and try to call. She meddled in the lives of her children to the point that she became physically sick from the stress it caused.

One day, after weeks of suggesting she leave her phone by her clothes so she could reap the benefits of massage, she finally agreed.   At first she got on the table without the phone but insisted the ringer be turned on. Within fifteen minutes the phone rang and her anxiety level rocketed. I thought she was going to blow up if I didn't give her that phone. The next week, we tried with the ringer off. She couldn't do it. It was as if the phone was heroin…

Things I Considered
- I wanted to yank the phone out of their hand.

- If I posted a huge sign on the massage room door that read, "NO PHONES BEYOND THIS POINT", maybe some people would actually oblige.

What I Did
I figured it's their massage. If they do not want to heed my advice then that's their prerogative. I've done my job by informing them how to receive the type of massage they requested.

What Not to Do
- When their phone rings, do not "accidentally" drop and crush their phone with your foot as you try to hand the device to your client.

- When your client asks you to please hand you their phone laying by their clothing, do not answer with an abrupt, "no." It comes across as rude. If they want to interact with their phone, that's their business.

TIPS

- Try not to entertain the reasons why they should be off their phones in order to relax. Just do your job. They are paying you to massage.
- You can politely ask them to turn the phone off during a massage with or without an explanation.

Body Odor Blues

Only once in the twenty-five years of working in the massage industry, have I come across a client who emitted a stench so unbearable that I could not proceed with the session. The odor fumigated my tiny office and seeped into my brain to the point where I became lightheaded and foggy. At first, I wasn't sure if the odor came from the shoes or socks or clothing. Perhaps it was only the feet. A simple remedy of hot moist towels and essentials oils could fix the problem! It was not that simple. The more I massaged, the more it seemed the stench pushed off the skin of the entire body, into the air.

The client, a twenty-one year-old, quiet young lady, had only one massage with me prior to this event. Lauren was pregnant at the time and living with friends. This did not seem like the same woman.

Things I Considered
- If she's living with people, didn't they inform her of her body odor?

- A discovery of a new treatment came to mind called

Full Body Steam Clean. This treatment uses steamed towels and essential oils to sterilize the entire body.

What I Did

Once my eyes started to burn and I started to cough, I knew I had a problem. When Lauren was prone and couldn't see me, I tried keeping my mouth and nose covered with my shirt but it was difficult to keep my head in a position where the shirt would stay on my face!

I had to discontinue the massage after a half hour. It was heroic of me to work on this person for that long!

After Lauren got dressed, I tried to tactfully discuss the reason why I cut the session short. I said, "Sometimes during a massage the lymph system moves substances out of the skin. For example the substances can be cigarettes, if you smoke or chemicals if you work with cleaning supplies. You are excreting something and it is too intoxicating for me to work on you. I'm sorry."

Lauren then told me her friend gave her the money for the massage and asked her to shower before she arrived, but she did not. She hadn't showered in months! Her postpartum depression was not getting better. It was worse.

Later, I learned the friend knew how much Lauren loved massages and hoped she would finally shower if she had an appointment.

What Not to Do

- Do not hold your breath in order not to choke on the intense odor.

- Don't cover your nose and chin with your shirt. It's too hard to keep the shirt on your face and massage at the same time. I tried it; it doesn't work!

TIPS

- Aromatherapy works well in covering or eliminating odors. Use essential oils in a diffuser or spray.

- Compliment the massage with a spa treatment: Keep a spray bottle of water with about 5-10 drops of lavender or peppermint. If the client isn't allergic or sensitive to essential oils, use directly on body as a mist. Spray a steamed towel and effleurage each arm, including the armpit, moving in a gentle flowing motion. Spray the arm again when the towels are removed. Massage the area. Repeat on all limbs and feet.

Request Your Free Templates

Holiday promotions, welcome cards, referral   cards and more.

Request your FREE templates from the book, *Successful Massage Business Marketing*, by Nina Ward. Also available on Amazon.

Email nina@ninawardwrites.com. Enter *FREE TEMPLATES* in subject line.

Feel free to contact me with any questions, feedback on this book, or just to say hello. Wishing you much success in your career.

ninawardwrites.com

Other Books

Successful Massage Business Guidebook, Nina Ward
Amazon https://www.amazon.com/dp/B07HNH7446

Hope for Recovery,
Stories of Healing from Eating Disorders
by Catherine Brown, Christina Tinker
Contributor, Nina Ward

www.ingramcontent.com/pod-product-compliance
Lightning Source LLC
Chambersburg PA
CBHW070808250726
48662CB00004B/2025